Quality of Care

A process for making
strategic choices in
health systems

WHO Library Cataloguing-in-Publication Data

Quality of care : a process for making strategic choices in health systems.

1.Quality assurance, Health care. 2.Health services administration. 3.Decision making. I. World Health Organization.

ISBN 92 4 156324 9   (NLM classification: W 84.1)
ISBN 978 92 4 156324 6

Printed in France

Contents

Acknowledgements

The World Health Organization (WHO) expresses appreciation to all those who contributed to the production of this document.

The authors and project team:
- Rafael Bengoa and Rania Kawar, Department of Health System Policies and Operations, WHO, Geneva
- Peter Key, Dearden Consulting Limited, United Kingdom
- Sheila Leatherman, University of North Carolina, USA and Judge Business School, University of Cambridge, United Kingdom
- Rashad Massoud, Institute for Healthcare Improvement, Cambridge, MA, USA
- Pedro Saturno, University of Murcia, Spain.

The core technical group included Ahmed Abdul Latif, Michael Adelhardt, Rebecca Bailey, Venkatraman Chandra-Mouli, Katie Edwards, Andrei Issakov, Rolf Korte, Itziar Larizgoitia, Hernan Montenegro, Anselm Schneider, Paul Van Ostenberg, Martin Weber, and Stuart Whittaker.

Valuable input and advice were provided by Sandra Black, Alimata Diarra-Nama, Christine Dowse, Enrique Terol Garcia, Maimunah Hamid, Graham Harrison, Khaled Hassan, Dale Huntington, Tom Mboya Okeyo, Hugo Mercer, Henock Alois Mayombo Ngonyani, Sue Page, Zinta Podniece, Sarah Prendergast, Osama Samawi, Maria Santos Ichaso, Tin Tin Sint, Sangay Thinley, Naruo Uehara, Mukund Uplekar, Orlando Urroz, Guillermo Williams, and Jelka Zupan.

Administrative and secretarial support was provided by Margaret Inkoom and Melanie McCallum.

Editing by Creative Publications

Graphic design and layout: Inís (www.inis.ie)

Foreword

This document provides decision-makers and managers at country level with a systematic process which will allow them to design and implement effective interventions to promote quality in health systems.

Conceived as a capacity-building tool in health-care quality, this guide focuses particular attention on people who have a strategic responsibility for quality. The reason for this approach is the understanding that in most countries there is an enormous amount of local readiness and action for quality improvement but frequently this action is carried out in an insufficient policy and strategic environment.

Furthermore, the process suggested here will help managers and decision-makers decide on which components of quality they wish to focus. In some countries, there may be more leverage for quality in reorganizing the delivery of care across settings, while in others it may be more appropriate to start with patient-safety activities. The intention, therefore, has been to keep the process simple and to avoid suggesting that 'one size fits all' and that there are 'magic bullets' for quality.

The guide also assumes that a common process of decision-making for policy-makers has relevance for the vast majority of countries, regardless of their particular circumstances. This assumption is made on the grounds that a robust process of decision-making will take into account country-specific factors – such as current resourcing, cultural sensitivity, affordability, and sustainability – in determining which combination of quality interventions will deliver the best outcomes and benefits for a country. The principles of quality management are largely identical across all countries, as they build on optimal use of scarce resources, client orientation, and sound planning, as well as evidence for improved quality of services.

Despite these commonalities across all countries, capacity-building in low- and middle-income countries has some specificities since it operates in a highly dynamic development context. During past decades, support to low- and middle-income countries has been driven by a supplier mentality. The focus was on the transfer of financial and physical resources and technology, with the assumption that this would trigger improvement. In many ways this supply-led logic continues to dominate in quality improvement – with a wide array of ready-made methods and brands being recommended to receptive health systems in low- and middle-income nations. Although many of these quality brands are very useful improvement approaches, this document is conceived to support countries in developing their own comprehensive strategies for quality before deciding to use specific branded approaches developed in other regions.

Recognizing the need to build capacity within countries, this guide has been designed to assist self-assessment and serve as a discussion guide so that decision-makers and interested parties in the quality arena can work together on finding answers for their own setting. The role of donors, development agencies, and/or consultant groups will be to support the implementation of these country-specific designs – not to substitute for them.

Rafael Bengoa

World Health Organization, Geneva
2006

Structure of the document

This guide is divided into the following four sections.

▨ Section 1, *Background and assumptions*, presents the context and rationale for developing this process.

▨ Section 2, *Basic concepts in quality*, provides simple working definitions of what is meant by quality in the context of health and health care, and describes various roles and responsibilities which apply to quality improvement in any health system.

▨ Section 3, *A process for building a strategy for quality: choosing interventions*, describes a decision-making process for policy-makers, which includes seven elements related to initial analysis, strategy development, and implementation. Within Element 5 of the decision-making process, special emphasis has been given to describing the various interventions for quality in the six principal domains.

▨ Section 4, *Annexes*, provides two tools:
  A. A self-assessment questionnaire for detailed analysis of Element 5 of the decision-making process.
  B. A matrix to map quality interventions by the various roles and responsibilities in a health system.

1. Background and assumptions

Why a focus on quality now?

A wealth of knowledge and experience in enhancing the quality of health care has accumulated globally over many decades. In spite of this wealth of experience, the problem frequently faced by policy-makers at country level in both high- and low-middle-income countries is to know which quality strategies – complemented by and integrated with existent strategic initiatives – would have the greatest impact on the outcomes delivered by their health systems. This guide promotes a focus on quality in health systems, and provides decision-makers and planners with an opportunity to make informed strategic choices to advance quality improvement.

There are two main arguments for promoting a focus on quality in health systems at this time.

- Even where health systems are well developed and resourced, there is clear evidence that quality remains a serious concern, with expected outcomes not predictably achieved and with wide variations in standards of health-care delivery within and between health-care systems.
- Where health systems – particularly in developing countries – need to optimize resource use and expand population coverage, the process of improvement and scaling up needs to be based on sound local strategies for quality so that the best possible results are achieved from new investment.

Why a focus on health systems and decision-makers?

The process in this document consciously addresses quality from a health-systems perspective. The rationale for doing so is best summarized in a quotation from an Institute of Medicine (USA) report[1]:

---

1 *Crossing the Quality Chasm: A New Health System for the 21st Century.* Committee on Quality of Health Care in America, Institute of Medicine. Washington, DC, USA: National Academies Press; 2001

As medical science and technology has advanced at a rapid pace, the health care delivery system has floundered in its ability to provide consistently high quality care to all.

This implies that increased know-how and increased resources will not, in themselves, translate into the high quality of health care which populations and individuals rightly expect. How one organizes the delivery of care has become as important. Health expenditure in industrialized countries has doubled in the last 30 years; however, the highest-spending countries are not always those with the best results.[2] One reason is the fragmentation of their health care delivery systems. Taking a systems perspective, and orienting systems to the delivery and improvement of quality, are fundamental to progress and to meeting the expectations of both populations and health-care workers.

Furthermore, achieving the Millennium Development Goals (MDGs) in low-income countries will also require an organized whole-system perspective. It is well recognized today that many low-income countries will have substantial difficulties in achieving the MDGs. The lack of sufficient financial investment, the fragmentation of the delivery of health services, and poor quality are considered key obstacles to the successful implementation of health programmes. A reflection of this is shown in recent studies in Pakistan, Sri Lanka, and the United Republic of Tanzania indicating that poor people bypass local services perceived as having lower quality, and instead access geographically distant public services or even incur costs by going to the private sector.[3] This practice may actually aggravate poverty.

In the recent past, there has been a steep increase in international development aid which is frequently organized via disease-specific programmes in international organizations or by the creation of new global health alliances and partnerships. There are at present more than 70 global health partnerships. Many of these initiatives have brought considerable improvement in countries. However, these initiatives have also brought some challenges. These challenges are mainly related to the coordination of fragmented, parallel efforts and to the lack of technical assistance which should accompany such new and ambitious financial support. Again the organized delivery of health care will be a key component to cope with the increasing verticality of projects in countries.

Within broader-sector plans being designed in countries, there is a growing understanding that health-system strengthening should become a priority in

---

2 Leatherman S, Sutherland K. Quality of care in the NHS of England. *British Medical Journal,* 2004, 328:E288–E290.

3 World Development Report. *Making services work for the poor.* Washington, DC, World Bank, 2004.

its own right. As this trend towards health-system strengthening increases, the strengthening of quality will become a key component which requires reform.

For this reason, the core focus of this document is on helping national and regional decision-makers and managers choose effective strategic interventions. However, the development of more coherent strategies for quality at country level should also enhance the capacity of local organizations delivering health care (hospitals, primary health-care centres), and that of the communities served, to improve quality outcomes.

Improving quality and whole-system reform

In every country, there is opportunity to improve the quality and performance of the health-care system, as well as growing awareness and public pressure to do so.

The decision-making process proposed in section 3 is intended to help decision-makers and managers work through a systematic process which leads towards selecting specific interventions to enhance quality and to improve outcomes and benefits for individuals and populations. The process encourages decision-makers to undertake a comprehensive situational analysis, and to revisit health goals and quality objectives before determining any new quality interventions.

Working through the process will create a new agenda for change, which focuses on improving the quality of the health system. The scope of that agenda cannot be anticipated for each application, and will always be the result of judgements and decisions of specific countries. In some cases, the selected interventions will serve to accelerate a process of improvement which is already in progress, and will build on existing systems and organizational models.

In other examples, the emerging programme of change might involve a more fundamental reorientation of the whole health system. This could include changes in how the health system is financed; in the system of remuneration of service providers; in the ownership of health-care delivery organizations; in systems of accountability; and in models of care. Large-scale change of this sort is often understood as "whole-system reform".

Thus, the issue for policy-makers and managers is to be aware that working through this decision-making process *may highlight the need for fundamental reform* in their health system. For example, issues of accessibility and equity, which are two dimensions of quality, are system dependent and can hardly be improved without reforming the broader system. Other dimensions of quality, such as patient safety, may not require broad reforms in order to move forward.

Sources of reassurance for policy-makers are that they control the use of the process, that the process deliberately involves a wide range of stakeholders, and that a natural consensus concerning the scale of change needed in the health system may well emerge.

Policy-making and evidence

There is a growing field of research concerning evidence for quality. This research reinforces a more scientific and systematic approach to the use of information concerning interventions on quality. The intention of this document is not to review the evidence across all the domains of quality, but rather to indicate to those who use this self-assessment guide where they may identify some key sources of evidence in those components of most interest to them.

These sources will help decision-makers seek information and draw upon the published evidence of the effectiveness and impact of various approaches to quality improvement which have been applied and evaluated – both in health care and more widely in other sectors.

However, it is important to highlight to users that the existing information on evidence of quality interventions in health care may be presented as neutral and as guidance that might be considered indicative of what works in general everywhere. It is important to emphasize that, in the field of quality, the context in which the evidence is being used is very important – the evidence cannot be considered to be as neutral as the evidence which is used, for example, in clinical decision-making.

Consequently it is important to keep in mind the following points.

- The general evidence-based information on quality is growing, and will increasingly be used – together with other deliberative processes – to inform decision-making in a process such as the self-assessment guide presented in this document. This is a very positive trend.
- Results are contextual, and evidence requires local interpretation by those involved in planning for quality. Diversity in practice makes published evidence heavily contextual. For example, the use of accreditation in various countries does not follow a standardized methodology, and therefore the results achieved by each country are not always directly comparable. Likewise,

new trends in patient safety (requiring de-emphasis of the entrenched hierarchy among various categories of health professionals) will be heavily contextual and very different among countries.

- Transferability of learning and experience is contextual. It cannot be assumed, for example, that a positive experience of quality improvement in one setting can be fully replicated in another where there are major cultural differences.
- The learning cycles implied in the various tools in this guide constitute in themselves a process for continued evaluation and improvement which – together with new evidence – provide increasing confidence for decision-makers.
- The above implies that policy-makers and managers who use the evidence from these sources will need to heavily contextualize the existing 'general' evidence within their own setting during their work on planning for quality. Policy-makers will need to exercise considerable judgement when making informed decisions about future quality interventions, and build dynamic processes which tailor local solutions and take into account new evidence as it arises.

Some of the sources on evidence include The Health Foundation (United Kingdom) which has commissioned a major research initiative (QQuIP) to analyse quality and efficiency in the National Health Service.[4] Within this initiative, there is a specific stream of work called Quality Enhancing Interventions (QEI). The QEI component is progressively releasing reports on impact which offer a series of structured reviews covering a wide range of possible interventions on quality. There are presently two reports available, one on the evidence of the impact of regulation on quality,[5] and the other on the effectiveness of patient-focused interventions.[6] Another key resource for evidence is the Agency for Healthcare Research and Quality.[7] In this source, decision-makers will find a set of evidence reports.

---

4 More on this initiative is available on http://www.health.org.uk/qquip

5 Sutherland K, Leatherman S. *Evidence of the impact of regulation on quality*. Quality Enhancing Interventions Project. (Working Paper 2006).

6 Coulter A, Ellins J. *The effectiveness of patient-focused interventions*. 2006.

7 http://www.ahrq.gov/

2. Basic concepts of quality

Definitions and the dimensions of quality

Every initiative taken to improve quality and outcomes in health systems has as its starting point some understanding of what is meant by 'quality'. Without this understanding, it would be impossible to design the interventions and measures used to improve results.

There are many definitions of quality used both in relation to health care and health systems, and in other spheres of activity. There is also a language of quality, with its own frequently-used terms.

For the purposes of this document, a working definition is needed to characterize quality in health care and health systems. Without such a working definition, the process of selecting new interventions and building strategies for quality improvement would be seriously impaired.

The focus of this guide is on health systems as a whole, and on the quality of the outcomes they produce. For this reason, this working definition needs to take a whole-system perspective, and reflect a concern for the outcomes achieved for both individual service users and whole communities.

The following working definition is used throughout the remainder of the document. It suggests that a health system should seek to make improvements in six areas or dimensions of quality, which are named and described below. These dimensions require that health care be:
- *effective*, delivering health care that is adherent to an evidence base and results in improved health outcomes for individuals and communities, based on need;
- *efficient*, delivering health care in a manner which maximizes resource use and avoids waste;
- *accessible*, delivering health care that is timely, geographically reasonable, and provided in a setting where skills and resources are appropriate to medical need;

- *acceptable/patient-centred*, delivering health care which takes into account the preferences and aspirations of individual service users and the cultures of their communities;
- *equitable*, delivering health care which does not vary in quality because of personal characteristics such as gender, race, ethnicity, geographical location, or socioeconomic status;
- *safe*, delivering health care which minimizes risks and harm to service users.

Roles and responsibilities in quality improvement

Another way to think about quality in health systems is to differentiate among roles, responsibilities in the various parts of a system.

The main concern of this document is to support the role of **policy and strategy development.** This critical activity will need to engage the whole health system, but lead responsibilities will normally rest at national and regional levels. The main concerns of decision-makers at these levels will be to keep the performance of the whole system under review, and to develop strategies for improving quality outcomes which apply across the whole system.

The core responsibilities of **health-service providers** for quality improvement are different. Providers may be seen as whole organizations, teams, or individual health workers. In each case, they will ideally be committed to the broad aims of quality policy for the whole system, but their main concern will be to ensure that the services they provide are of the highest possible standard and meet the needs of individual service users, their families, and communities.

Improved quality outcomes are not, however, delivered by health-service providers alone. **Communities and service users** are the co-producers of health. They have critical roles and responsibilities in identifying their own needs and preferences, and in managing their own health with appropriate support from health-service providers.

While it is important to recognize these differences in roles and responsibilities, it is equally important to recognize the connections between them. Examples include the following.

- Decision-makers cannot hope to develop and implement new strategies for quality without properly engaging health-service providers, communities, and service users.

10

- Health-service providers need to operate within an appropriate policy environment for quality, and with a proper understanding of the needs and expectations of those they serve, in order to deliver the best results.
- Communities and service users need to influence both quality policy and the way in which health services are provided to them, if they are to improve their own health outcomes.

These critical relationships are summarized in Figure 1.

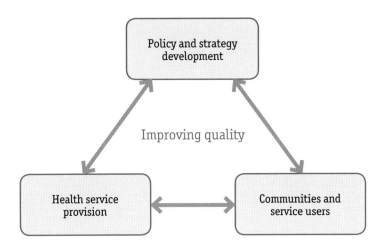

Figure 1: *Roles and responsibilities in quality improvement*

3. A process for building a strategy for quality: choosing interventions

An overview of the suggested process

This section proposes an approach for decision-making at country level, to make informed strategic interventions for predictable quality improvement.

This suggested approach is meant only as a guideline. In reality, any process of policy-making at country level has to be determined locally and to take full account of local circumstances and preferences. The first step in applying the process in any country would therefore be to agree whether this approach needs to be modified to fit the local situation better. Nevertheless, ensuring that every element of the process is addressed will facilitate a comprehensive approach to quality improvement across the health system.

The process is deliberately simple, and does not propose any activity which will be unfamiliar to policy-makers. It is based on the practical experience of governments and development organizations making informed choices about how to advance a quality improvement agenda in health.

The suggested process, presented in Figure 2, is cyclical. It contains seven activities ("elements") within the three categories of **analysis**, **strategy**, and **implementation**. As a cyclical process it reflects a frequently adopted approach to quality improvement – understand the problem, plan, take action, study the results, and plan new actions in response. The main implication of this approach is that strategies for quality improvement are not 'fixed'. While the broad direction of progress may be consistent, responding to results will always require that adaptations be made to some elements of the strategy and to the approach for implementation.

There is a danger that the suggested process will be interpreted as needing extended timescales for the early stages of analysis and decision-making. Experience in the field suggests that this need not be the case. As long as the process is well planned, appropriately resourced, and driven by available information as well as active stakeholder participation, an agreed quality-improvement strategy could be produced in a short period.

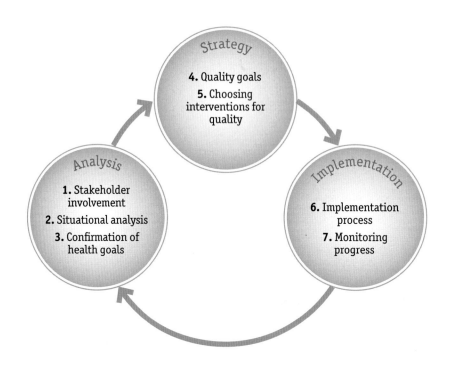

Figure 2: *A process for building a strategy for quality*

Analysis

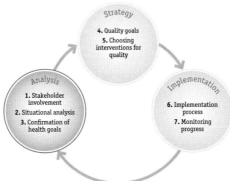

This first part of the cyclical process of strategy development and implementation has three elements. These elements are all significant and they interact. However, the entry point for decision-makers into this part of the process could be at any of the three elements.

Element 1. **Stakeholder involvement**

Quality improvement is about change. For this reason, an important early step in the decision-making process is to determine who are the key stakeholders and how they will be involved.

Key stakeholders would normally include political and community leaders, service users and their advocates, health-care delivery organizations, regulatory bodies, and representative bodies for health workers. A further central group of stakeholders would be the senior officials responsible for quality within the ministry of health. Depending on how such responsibilities are allocated, there may be several policy leaders addressing different aspects of quality.

A key method of involvement could be the formation of a board or steering group drawn from the stakeholder groups, that would remain involved in all stages of the process, including implementation and the review of progress. The board or steering group could provide the main focus for accountability and preparing advice to decision-makers, as well as wider communication with all interested parties. Clear terms of reference would be essential.

To avoid confusion, those leading the process would need to know clearly from the outset who would make policy decisions and determine the range of new quality interventions.

The following questions may, therefore, be useful to decision-makers as they analyse stakeholder involvement.

- Is there a clear process for involving stakeholders?
- Is there a list of all key stakeholders?
- Are there clear terms of reference for all interested parties?

Element 2. **Situational analysis**

Choosing new interventions for quality improvement in a health system will always take place against a background of existing policies and priorities, as well as current health-system performance. These factors cannot be ignored, and need to be part of the thinking process. For this reason, a critical part of the cycle is to conduct a situational analysis.

Situational analysis is a mapping process which allows a clear baseline to be established before any new interventions are considered or existing ones adapted. While the main focus of the situational analysis is on the health system, it also needs to make connections between health and other sectors and issues which will impact on the performance of the health system.

The situational analysis will need to cover many areas, which might include the following.

- Current structures and systems within the ministry of health relating to quality improvement. Does there exist clear leadership and accountability, and is quality managed in an integrated way at the centre or is there a problem of fragmentation?
- Current policies in health and across sectors (e.g. where there are national policies for quality which apply to all sectors, including health). The aim would be to fully understand the quality implications of those policies as well as to search out the degree of alignment, policy themes and obstacles, and opportunities that follow from the current national policy agenda. This applies to both government and professional policies.
- Current health goals and priorities. The aim here would be to understand the nature of those goals and priorities, how they are being addressed, and particularly the contribution that quality improvement is making to their achievement.
- Current performance of the health system. How does the system perform overall, and particularly against the dimensions of quality? Is health care effective, efficient, accessible, acceptable, equitable, and safe? How does the

payment system influence quality? How does the performance compare with that of other countries with similar circumstances? The purpose of this stage of the process is not to overanalyse the health system in a country, but rather simply to obtain a general description of health-system performance. Those who wish to investigate further the current performance of their health system may wish to use a set of both process and outcome measures that are designed to compare the quality of various health systems.[8]

- Current quality interventions. How is the system acting now in the various domains of quality improvement? What effect is there on information, leadership, engagement with patients and the population, the use of regulation and standards, developing organizational capacity, and models of care? What impact are those current activities having on the quality of health care and on outcomes?

The success of the situational analysis in establishing a sound baseline understanding for the cycle of strategy development, implementation, and review will be determined by:

- the availability of analyst time to collect – on behalf of the steering group – required information from a wide range of sources, both national and international;
- the willingness of the steering group to work with existing and easily accessed data, rather than generating new information requirements at this stage (which will slow down the process);
- the willingness of the steering group to work with perceptions (and especially service-user perceptions) as well as with quantitative information.

Element 3. Confirmation of health goals

The third element in the process of analysis is to confirm the wider health goals of the health system. This activity is included as a separate element because:

- it will be critical for any new interventions in quality improvement to be seen by stakeholders as aligned with and serving the broader health goals of the system;
- the situational analysis may cause some health goals to be called into question by policy-makers and other stakeholders;
- without clear and agreed health goals, the focus and purpose of any new quality intervention is questionable.

---

8 Kelley E, Hurst J. *Health care quality indicators project*. Paris, Organisation for Economic Co-operation and Development, 2006 (OECD Health Working Papers, No. 23). This OECD project uses the same multidimensional framework for quality that is used in this document.

In the case of the last of these three situations, the process of decision-making about quality needs to be held in abeyance until there is certainty and clarity about health goals.

The health goals of any health system will normally be set through a political process, and may be wide-ranging. They might fall within the following broad categories.

- *Reducing mortality:* for example, aiming to increase life expectancy for the population as a whole or for groups within the population (e.g. children).
- *Reducing morbidity:* for example, aiming to reduce the incidence of a particular disease such as malaria or diabetes, within the population.
- *Reducing health inequalities:* for example, aiming to narrow the gap in life expectancy between different social groups within the wider population.
- *Improving outcomes for a particular disease:* for example, improving survival rates for people with cancer or AIDS.
- *Making health care safer:* for example, reducing the incidence and impact of hospital acquired infections.

Building the strategy: Choosing interventions for quality

The second part of the cyclical process is concerned with the development of new strategies in response to analysis, the selection of appropriate interventions, and planning for their implementation. This process is divided into two elements.

Element 4. Development of quality goals

With health goals and priorities confirmed, and a situational analysis completed, the ground is prepared for new quality goals to be negotiated and agreed. This will lead to the selection of quality interventions.

The choice of quality goals will be driven by the agreed health goals, and will relate to the different dimensions of quality. The questioning process in relation to the health goal will be to ask the following.

- What are the deficiencies in effectiveness?
- What are the deficiencies in efficiency?
- What are the deficiencies in accessibility?
- What are the deficiencies in acceptability?
- What are the deficiencies in equity?
- What are the deficiencies in safety?

In answering these questions, the evidence gathered in the situational analysis should be invaluable. In particular, the situational analysis should inform judgements about the significance of general evidence for a particular health issue. For example, there may be a general perception that access to health care is reasonable. There may also be evidence that delays in access to health care are affecting outcomes for particular populations.

The following examples illustrate the connections between broader health goals and related quality goals.

- *Health goal:* improve health outcomes for rural populations.
  Quality goals: improve local access to health services; improve the acceptability of those services.
- *Health goal:* reduce avoidable mortality from preventable risks.
  Quality goals: reduce medication errors by 50%.
- *Health goal:* improve outcomes for people with cancer.
  Quality goals: improve access to diagnostics and early treatment; improve effectiveness through evidence-based practice; ensure continuity of care.

In these examples, both the health goals and the related quality goals are expressed in very general terms. In practice, the steering group and other decision-makers would need to ensure that these goals were explicit, time-bound, and measurable, so that they would provide the basis for measuring progress and the impact of new interventions later in the change process.

Element 5. Choosing interventions for quality

The earlier elements in this suggested decision-making process focus on an analysis of the present situation, and on clearly defining priorities and goals. They are therefore very much about the "whats" of a change process. They also provide a critical component in any strategy for improvement – clarity about what the strategy is trying to achieve.

This element moves attention from the "what" to the "how". It calls for judgements to be made about interventions, and agreement to be reached about the process of implementation.

Mapping the domains

Having undergone an organized analysis of needs and a determination of health goals and quality goals, decision-makers need to work through the options for interventions in order to build a strategy on quality. To assist this process, it is helpful to follow a simple 'map' of the domains where quality interventions could be made (and where current quality problems might be located).

Figure 3 presents such a map. It identifies six domains which are generic in nature, and which are interrelated. They are intended to help policy-makers address quality issues at a more strategic level.

Figure 3: *The six domains of quality interventions*

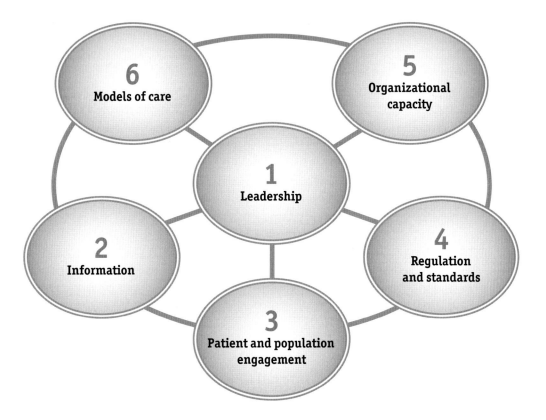

These generic domains are not hypothetical. They draw heavily on the strategies for quality improvement applied in many health systems over many decades. Many countries heavily emphasize only one domain (e.g. regulation) in their work on quality. The process in this document suggests that it is necessary to follow a more comprehensive approach across the several domains shown in the map.

The following descriptions of the domains do not claim to be comprehensive. The examples given of the issues and options are meant to be illustrative, and sufficient to inform a thinking process for decision-makers.

Domain 1. Leadership

Leadership is the first domain, and is at the heart of Figure 3 because the issues involved underpin the development of any coherent strategy for quality improvement.

Leadership is fundamental because there is clear evidence that quality initiatives fail to realize their desired outcomes if there is not strong and consistent leadership support – at every level – for the action being taken. In the absence of strong and sustained leadership across the health system, any new strategic interventions are therefore unlikely to succeed.

For the best outcomes to be achieved, strong leadership and support for quality needs to come from national and community leaders, as well as leaders of health-service delivery organizations.

Where there are perceived weaknesses in leadership in the health system, strategic interventions may be needed to build commitment and leadership capacity, and to strengthen accountability.

Domain 2. Information

Information is fundamental, because any quality improvement is dependent on the capacity to measure change in processes and outcomes, and on stakeholders having access to the information that changes what they do.

To be fully effective, information systems for quality improvement need to apply consistently across the whole system, so that comparisons in outcomes and progress can be made between parts of the system. Those systems also need to be transparent, so that the widest possible range of stakeholders has access to the same information.

Information systems which support quality improvement can be complex and resource-intensive. One of the commitments needed from leaders is to ensure that a proper level of investment in information systems is maintained. Improvements need not depend on high-tech information technology. In some countries, fairly simple information systems – such as sheets with boxes to tick the basic processes of good child care – may be very valuable as decision-support systems. In other countries, computer prompts may be possible.

The scope of the information domain includes the availability to health workers of information about best practice; the way in which information is given to service users by those providing care; and the access by communities and individuals to information which will help them manage their own health. Any of these areas might require change as part of a strategy for quality improvement.

Domain 3. Patient and population engagement

The third domain is engagement with patients and the population. This domain is critical to quality improvement, because individuals and communities play so many roles within health systems. Either directly or indirectly, they will be financing care, they will be working in partnership with health workers to manage their own care, and they will sometimes be the final arbiter of what is acceptable and what is not across all the dimensions of quality.

The challenge to health systems is to ensure that engagement with patients and the population is at the heart of all policies and strategies for quality improvement, and that this commitment is translated into meaningful action. Strategies to this end include those which target improving health literacy, self-care, and patients' experience with the health system. Communities and service users will want to be involved in the governance arrangements of the health system; they will want their views and preferences to be heard and taken into account in decision-making; and they will want to share the responsibility for their own health. New strategic interventions in quality may be needed to realize these aspirations.

Domain 4. Regulation and standards

The fourth domain, regulation and standards, is frequently visited in the quest for quality improvement in health systems and offers considerable scope for policy interventions at country level. Inspection and accreditation at varying levels can be provided as appropriate to the resources available in the country. Setting standards and monitoring adherence to them may be one of the more efficient means of facilitating higher compliance with evidence.

23

That scope is not limited by the fundamental characteristics of the health system (e.g. by the system of funding for health care, or by the level of government involvement in the delivery of health services), because of the power to legislate and regulate which is held by all governments. It is, however, a domain in which professional bodies and regulatory agencies for health workers will often play a major part – either independently or in partnership with governments.

The use of regulation and standards seeks to change performance through the application of externally developed measures. Their use by health-service providers is often subject to external inspection or accreditation, and contrasts with other approaches to quality improvement which are more internally driven. The challenge to policy-makers is to find the right balance between internal and external drivers for improvement, and reflect that balance in their strategy for quality.

Domain 5. Organizational capacity

The fifth domain involves organizational capacity. The issues for quality in this domain apply throughout the health system. At the national level, there should be the capacity to lead the development of policy, to drive implementation, and to keep performance under review. Within communities, there should be the capacity to identify needs and preferences and to articulate them within the health system. Issues of capacity are, however, particularly relevant for those organizations which are delivering health services to individuals and communities – as this is the interface at which users directly experience the quality of care available to them.

Whether a health-service-provider organization is in the government sector, the private sector, or is part of a nongovernmental organization, the capacity issues on which they need to focus in order to deliver quality to service users remain the same. They will mainly be concerned with their ability to develop systems to support quality improvement such as audit and peer-review; their capacity to develop their workforce and equip them with the skills needed to deliver quality; their ability to build an organizational culture which values quality; and their ability to use rewards and incentives to promote that culture.

Domain 6. Models of care

The final domain reflects currently understood best practice for the delivery of health care generically and to particular population groups, such as groups defined by a common need (e.g. people with chronic conditions) or common characteristics (e.g. children or the elderly).

The development of new models of care will normally aim to address all the dimensions of quality described earlier (i.e. effective, efficient, accessible, acceptable/patient-centred, equitable, and safe) and will seek to improve outcomes by organizing integrated responses.

The development of models of care is differentiated from organizational capacity because when health systems focus on models of care to improve quality, they will normally find themselves working beyond individual institutions and therefore working across the boundaries of health-care organizations and with large population bases. In other words, in order to improve quality, it is necessary to focus on the delivery system as a whole.

A new model of care may need to integrate the contributions of primary, specialized, and social care organizations. This new model should span the whole continuum of care – including health promotion and protection – in order to improve quality outcomes. It is important for decision-makers to consider that the reorganization of health care across settings, and seeking integrated and continuous care may provide the largest leverage in quality improvement. For example, the use of The Chronic Care Model – which seeks quality improvement and better management of chronic conditions – is one approach to more continuous care.[9]

The development of new models of care usually involves high levels of stakeholder involvement (including service users and communities), an appraisal of evidence, the development of protocols and guidelines, and a process to redesign the delivery of care. The challenge to policy-makers is to know when this approach is needed, and for which population groups.

Linking the domains to the decision-making process

As seen in Figure 4, the domains are mainly useful for Element 5 of the process, particularly for choosing the specific strategic interventions on quality. Annex A provides an expanded array of questions to help planners explore each domain in more detail.

---

9 Wagner EH. Chronic disease management. What will it take to improve care for chronic illness? *Effective Clinical Practice*, 1998, 1:2–4.

Figure 4: *Linking the domains to the decision-making process*

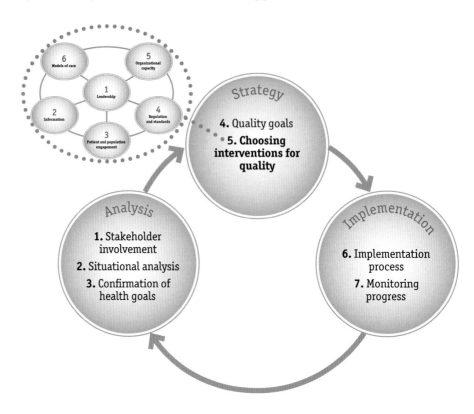

Deciding on interventions

Determining the "how" means selecting those interventions in quality which will deliver the improved outcomes and benefits being sought. Again, the situational analysis should provide a helpful baseline for making those judgements. For instance, a leadership intervention may be needed to address poorly aligned or conflicting policies which were identified at that stage. Alternatively, the situational analysis may have identified weaknesses in engagement with patients and the population which could undermine interventions to improve outcomes for patients with a particular disease.

The framework of domains for quality interventions suggested above is intended as a simple prompt for decision-makers. It is likely that most domains will need reinforcement in one way or another. However, when the framework is used systematically – in relation to any of the agreed goals – it invites identification of the domains on which decision-makers need to focus and prioritize at this particular time in the process. Again, these domains are as follows.

1. Leadership
2. Information
3. Patient and population engagement
4. Regulation and standards
5. Organizational capacity
6. Models of care.

Another important outcome to be achieved in this part of the cycle is agreement about the plan for implementation of the agreed interventions. Any implementation plan will need to meet local considerations, but there are generic issues which need to be considered, such as those suggested in the following questions.

- Who will lead the change process?
- What resources will be available to support implementation?
- What technical expertise will be available to support implementation?
- How will accountability work?
- Who has the authority to amend the implementation plan?
- Will the change process start with pilot projects?
- What will be the plan for scaling up?
- What will be the timetable for implementation?
- How will decision-makers communicate with stakeholders?
- What will be the key milestones?
- How will progress be monitored?

Agreement on these various issues will establish a quality-improvement strategy with the following main elements.

- Quality goals derived from agreed health goals.
- Selected interventions in various quality domains, which are most likely to deliver the desired improvements.
- A detailed plan for managing the implementation of those interventions.

Implementation......

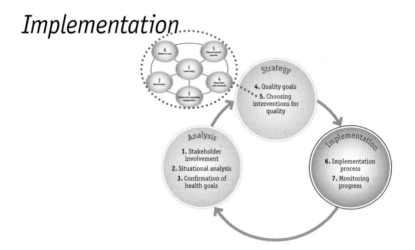

The third part of the cyclical process is concerned with the management of agreed quality strategies, and with reviewing progress and the impact of changes as an input to the continuing activity of ANALYSIS.

Element 6. Implementation process

The production of an agreed quality-improvement strategy is still a very early stage in the process of change. This element moves the focus to managing the implementation process. The strategy will have identified a framework for implementation and covered key issues such as leadership and accountability, timescales and milestones, and the monitoring of progress.

The success of the interventions will then depend on maintaining a clear focus on implementation, sustaining interest and commitment, and having the capacity to make tactical decisions to modify activities in response to feedback. All of this is critical for sustainability, as many quality-improvement initiatives encounter declining results because they lack sustained focus on implementation.

Having a programme board or steering group with appropriate stakeholder representation and terms of reference could be an effective way of sustaining a focus on and interest in the implementation of the quality improvement strategy. The core responsibilities of such a board might include:
- keeping under review progress on implementation, adherence to timetables, and achievement of targets and goals;
- redirecting resources;
- providing an account of progress to interested parties;
- modifying timetables and milestones;

- preparing the health system for scaling up where a phased approach is planned;
- keeping new evidence under review and modifying plans to take account of that evidence.

The programme board or steering group would also have a major leadership role within the change process, which would include:
- promoting the shared vision of the future for improved quality, both within the health system and more widely with stakeholders;
- continuing to challenge the status quo;
- empowering others to act on their behalf – for example, forming teams for each strategy to undertake specific tasks;
- offering encouragement and celebrating progress and success.

Element 7. Monitoring progress

The final element is to maintain a focus on the delivery of the improved outcomes and benefits being sought. This focus is important because:
- if results are not those that were expected, it will be important to make early decisions about how the strategy and its selected interventions might be modified to achieve better results;
- any investment of effort and resources in quality improvement can only be justified in terms of improved outcomes – giving proper account to stakeholders for that investment can only be done with information about changing outcomes; and
- maintaining the motivation and commitment of stakeholders in the change process will be helped by being able to point both to progress and achievements, and to the delivery of the quality goals to which they have subscribed.

The quality measures to be used will have been agreed earlier in the process, when health goals and related quality goals were set. Wherever possible, existing information sources should be used to monitor progress and outcomes; the implementation plan should include arrangements for collecting new data if required.

Experience with change processes and the development of supporting information systems suggest that:
- stakeholders should be actively involved in the design of any new system;
- new information systems should be made as simple as possible e.g. through the use of sampling techniques;

- any new information system should have local operational value, as well as serving the need to monitor changing outcomes at the national level; and
- the introduction of new systems should be supported with appropriate staff orientation and training.

The most important contribution of a continuing process of monitoring will be in completing the cycle of ANALYSIS, STRATEGY and IMPLEMENTATION. Completing this cycle will in turn provide the feedback which will allow elements of the strategy – and of plans for implementation – to be modified.

ANNEX A:
A self-assessment questionnaire for detailed analysis of Element 5 of the decision-making process

This self-assessment question-naire is offered as a tool for an expanded analysis of Element 5 of the decision-making process.

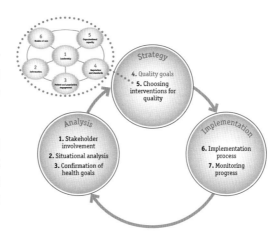

It attempts to cover a broad range of issues which might need to be considered in each of the six domains described in section 3.

The tool, as it is described here, is offered as a template. Before it is used by decision-makers, consideration should be given to modifying the content to best fit the particular circumstances of the country concerned.

Element 5. **Choosing interventions for quality**

Domain 1. Leadership

1. Are national leaders committed to improving quality in health systems?
2. Is there a clear system of leadership and accountability for quality which extends throughout the health system and which is not fragmented?
3. Are there processes and forums in place throughout the health system, which engage clinical and community leaders in developing policies and strategies for quality, and in reviewing progress?
4. Are leaders throughout the health system empowered to take action in pursuit of improved quality?

5. Are leadership development programmes provided throughout the health system to strengthen individual leadership skills and to enhance overall leadership capacity?

6. Are leaders in quality supported by an appropriate infrastructure and resources to facilitate their leadership activities?

7. Are leaders throughout the health system building a culture of excellence in pursuit of improved quality?

8. Are leaders throughout the health system interacting with communities, service users, and those who choose not to use services, in order to understand their needs and preferences?

9. Do leaders throughout the health system ensure that information about the quality of service provision and about quality outcomes is widely shared with stakeholders?

Domain 2. Information

10. Do existing information systems allow quality and performance to be monitored on a continuing basis across the health system?

11. Is the information so produced used to inform policy decisions in a systematic way?

12. Is information about quality and performance made widely available to interested parties, including patients and communities, as part of the general approach to quality improvement?

13. Do existing information systems have the capacity to respond to future demands in quality improvement?

14. Is there an appropriate investment in the human resources which are needed to maintain and operate information systems, and to analyse and interpret the information being produced?

15. Do all health workers have easy access to current evidence of best practice in their field?

16. Do health workers have appropriate access to expert systems which guide their practice?

17. Do health workers find it easy to pool information about patients whose care they share, across organizational boundaries and across a continuum of care?

18. Do health-service providers supply information to individual patients and carers in ways which maximize understanding?

19. Do individuals, families, and communities have easy access to information which will help them manage their own health?

20. Do the users of health services have sufficient information to enable them to make informed choices about how they use these services?

21. Are patient and population satisfaction surveys used across the health system to assess community and user perceptions of the quality of services being provided?
22. How does the national policy agenda on quality relate to marginalized groups and the poor?

Domain 3. Patient and population engagement

23. Are the rights of service users and communities at the heart of quality policy throughout the health system?
24. Are service users and communities properly involved in the governance of all parts of the health system?
25. Are service users and communities properly involved in systems of accreditation and in the governance of professional bodies?
26. Are individual users of services, and their families, appropriately involved with health workers in making shared decisions about their own care, and are these users and their families helped to make informed choices?
27. Is good health seen by individuals and communities as an outcome for which they share responsibility with the health system?

Domain 4. Regulation and standards

28. Across the health system, is there an appropriate balance between externally imposed standards, and processes of quality improvement which rely on self-regulation and peer review?
29. Are existing systems of regulation and standard setting kept under review, and is their impact on quality outcomes assessed?
30. When new standards and regulations are developed and introduced, do they reflect the goals and priorities of the health system?
31. Are all standards evidence-based and do they reflect normative guidance, adapted to the national context?
32. Are users of services, communities, and health workers all involved in the development of new standards and regulations?
33. Do systems of initial training and certification for health workers produce practitioners who are both competent and committed to quality?
34. Are systems of initial training and certification regularly reviewed and updated to reflect priorities for quality improvement?
35. Do processes of recertification for health workers reflect priorities for quality improvement?

36. Are processes of self-regulation for health workers built upon agreed standards of practice?

Domain 5. Organizational capacity

37. Is there capacity at the national level to focus attention on a quality agenda for the health system, and to deliver sustained leadership to the system?
38. Are health-service-provider organizations encouraged to develop their own strategies and procedures for quality improvement, within the context of national quality policy?
39. Within health-service-provider organizations, is local leadership and accountability for quality outcomes always clear?
40. Do health-service-provider organizations systematically promote a culture within which quality improvement is central to the purposes of the organization?
41. Do health-service-provider organizations regularly review those key systems which contribute to quality goals, including systems for managing risk and safety, systems for obtaining user views, and systems for training and education?
42. Do health-service-provider organizations systematically develop the capacity of their staff to analyze quality data, identify problems and manage change?
43. Are health-service-provider organizations providing continuing professional development for their staff to promote quality improvement?
44. Do health-service-provider organizations have the capacity to develop, maintain, and improve their information systems to support quality improvement?
45. Do health-service-provider organizations have the capacity to implement externally developed standards, protocols, and guidelines, and to monitor their use?
46. Do health-service-provider organizations have the capacity to design and implement their own protocols and guidelines?
47. Do health-service-provider organizations have the capacity to develop and implement new roles within their workforce?
48. Do health-service-provider organizations use incentives and rewards for individuals and teams, to promote quality improvement?
49. Do communities have the capacity and resources to identify and articulate their health needs and preferences?

Domain 6. Models of care

50. Is the reorganization of the delivery of health care perceived as a tool for quality improvement?
51. Are there mechanisms in place which allow new models of care to be developed with the full involvement of health-service providers, service users and communities?
52. Are new models of care developed in response to national priorities and health goals (e.g. for TB, cancer, children)?
53. Are new models of care evidence-based?
54. Do new models of care span across all aspects of health care, and do they integrate self-management by service users and the contributions of communities, as well as the contributions of health-service providers?
55. Are the models of care providing seamless and continuous care?
56. Is the implementation of new models of care always appropriately provided with resources?
57. Is the impact of models of care on quality outcomes kept under continuous review?

ANNEX B:
A matrix to map quality interventions by roles and responsibilities in a health system

Having chosen the interventions, it is interesting to show the extent to which each quality domain is being addressed by those interventions, as reflected in the following question. To what extent will the future quality programme include interventions in leadership, information, engagement with patients and the population, regulation and standards, organizational capacity, and models of care?

In order to continue the self-assessment process, the matrix below offers the possibility of locating the chosen interventions for each domain according to the various roles described in section 2. For example, the following questions can be asked within the context of this matrix.

- Which quality interventions are required to change the ways in which policy is made?
- Which interventions are needed in relation to service provision?
- Which interventions are needed to strengthen the contributions made by communities and service users?

Figure 5: *A matrix for mapping quality interventions at country level*

DOMAINS						
ROLES	Domain 1 Leadership	Domain 2 Information	Domain 3 Patient & population engagement	Domain 4 Regulation & standards	Domain 5 Organizational capacity	Domain 6 Models of care
Policy & strategy development						
Health service provision						
Communities & service users						

Given the high cost of some interventions for quality, it is relevant for countries to consider which are the main interventions they wish to implement to satisfy their overall health and quality goals. It may be unrealistic to invest in all the domains and levels of the matrix presented above. Policy-makers and managers would need to choose the interventions that they believe will achieve the biggest leverage. From these choices, the matrix would show the principal areas for intervention.